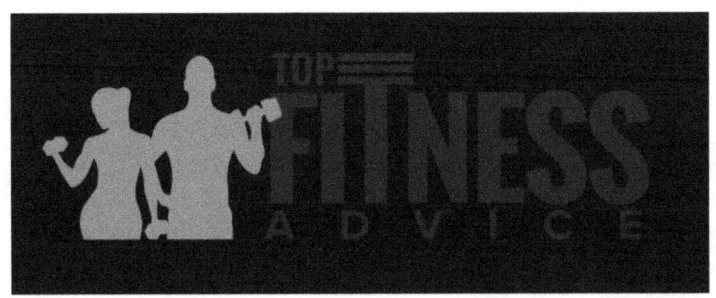

HEALTHY HABITS VOL. 1

The 13 Morning Habits That Can Help You To Lose Weight, Feel More Energized & Live A Healthier Life!

LINDA WESTWOOD

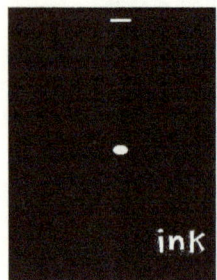

First published in 2015 by Venture Ink Publishing

Copyright © Top Fitness Advice 2019

All rights reserved.

No part of this book may be reproduced in any form without permission in writing from the author. No part of this publication may be reproduced or transmitted in any form or by any means, mechanic, electronic, photocopying, recording, by any storage or retrieval system, or transmitted by email without the permission in writing from the author and publisher.

Requests to the publisher for permission should be addressed to publishing@ventureink.co

For more information about the contents of this book or questions to the author, please contact Linda Westwood at linda@topfitnessadvice.com

Disclaimer

This book provides wellness management information in an informative and educational manner only, with information that is general in nature and that is not specific to you, the reader. The contents of this book are intended to assist you and other readers in your personal wellness efforts. Consult your physician regarding the applicability of any information provided in this book to you.

Nothing in this book should be construed as personal advice or diagnosis, and must not be used in this manner. The information provided about conditions is general in nature. This information does not cover all possible uses, actions, precautions, side-effects, or interactions of medicines, or medical procedures. The information in this book should not be considered as complete and does not cover all diseases, ailments, physical conditions, or their treatment.

You should consult with your physician before beginning any exercise, weight loss, or health care program. This book should not be used in place of a call or visit to a competent health-care professional. You should consult a health care professional before adopting any of the suggestions in this book or before drawing inferences from it.

Any decision regarding treatment and medication for your condition should be made with the advice and consultation of a qualified health care professional. If you have, or suspect you have, a health-care problem, then you should immediately contact a qualified health care professional for treatment.

No Warranties: The author and publisher don't guarantee or warrant the quality, accuracy, completeness, timeliness, appropriateness or suitability of the information in this book, or of any product or services referenced in this book.

The information in this book is provided on an "as is" basis and the author and publisher make no representations or warranties of any kind with respect to this information. This book may contain inaccuracies, typographical errors, or other errors.

Liability Disclaimer: The publisher, author, and other parties involved in the creation, production, provision of information, or delivery of this book specifically disclaim any responsibility, and shall not be held liable for any damages, claims, injuries, losses, liabilities, costs, or obligations including any direct, indirect, special, incidental, or consequences damages (collectively known as "Damages") whatsoever and howsoever caused, arising out of, or in connection with the use or misuse of the site and the information contained within it, whether such Damages arise in contract, tort, negligence, equity, statute law, or by way of other legal theory.

Table of Contents

Disclaimer 3

Who is this book for? 9

What will this book teach you? 11

Introduction 13

Morning Habit #1: The MOST Common Habit of Healthy People 15

Morning Habit #2: The Morning Drink That Will Change Your Life 23

Morning Habit #3: Get Your Blood Flowing 27

Morning Habit #4: Start Moving ASAP 31

Morning Habit #5: The BIGGEST Mistake Most People Make in The Morning 37

Morning Habit #6: Stack Your Breakfast With THIS 45

Morning Habit #7: A Morning Fat Burning Boost 49

Morning Habit #8: The Crucial Habit to Weight Loss Success 55

Morning Habit #9: The ONLY Pill That You Should Take 59

Morning Habit #10: Boost Your Fiber Intake 63

Morning Habit #11: The MOST Important Habit in This Book   67

Morning Habit #12: Plan to Be A Binge Drinker   69

Morning Habit #13: Make & Carry Healthy Snacks with You   73

BONUS Morning Habit #14: Carb Up in the AM!   75

BONUS Morning Habit #15: The Only OTHER Pill That You Should Take   77

BONUS Morning Habit #16: Rebound to A Healthy Life   79

Conclusion   85

Final Words   87

Would you prefer to listen to my book, rather than read it?

Download the audiobook version for free!

If you go to the special link below and sign up to Audible as a new customer, you can get the audiobook version of my book completely free.

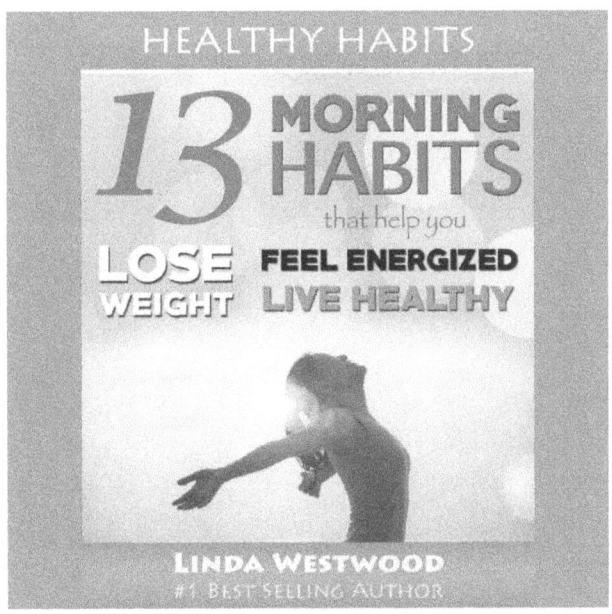

Go here to get your audiobook version for free:

TopFitnessAdvice.com/go/morning

Who is this book for?

Have you tried to lose weight before but failed?

Are you struggling to stick to healthy habits?

Are you one of those people who *know* what to do, but struggle to *actually do* it?

Then this book is for you!

I am going to share with you some of the MOST effective morning habits that you can add into your life to lose weight, feel great and be energized throughout your entire day!

I have given you a simple action plan at the end of each chapter so you can implement each habit very easily!

Also, you don't have to be overweight to benefit from these habits.

Yes, they help you lose weight, but they also help you live a healthy life, as well as feel recharged and energized ALL DAY LONG!

What will this book teach you?

This book is not like others!

It doesn't just contain generic advice that we all already know, but actual morning habits that have been identified to INCREASE weight loss, IMPROVE energy levels, and LEAD to a more healthy life!

Some of these habits are very simple and you can begin implementing them from tomorrow morning, and some are a little more difficult, in that you will need to practice them more!

I will also share with you why each of these habits work and are so effective – along with a simple action plan to help get you started and on your way to lasting success!

Introduction

Want to lose weight and feel great? Then this is the book for you.

If you are anything like me, you have tried just about every diet on the planet and have lost and regained weight several times over.

It's a vicious cycle – you diet and lose the fat, only to find that it arrives back with MORE when the diet is over!

Diets don't work! They create an unnatural feeling of deprivation and the body starts to rebel quite fast.

I, for example, am not a choc-a-holic – I enjoy chocolates, but don't eat too many of them… until I go on a diet.

Once I start a diet my body starts demanding chocolates, and all the other stuff I shouldn't be eating.

Many people find that the same type of thing happens to them. Dieting is clearly not the answer. If dieting did work, there would only be one diet plan out there and no one would be overweight or obese.

This book is different – it is not a diet book.

In this book, I'll give you 13 little habits that you can add into your lifestyle so that you naturally and painlessly lose weight and keep it off.

Thirteen may seem like a lot but here's the rub – you will adopt each one individually, at your own pace. In fact, I insist that you do not rush it – this process should take no less than two weeks at the very least.

I know that you are motivated to get started on everything now, but this program works because it is done step-by-step. Introducing each habit individually allows your body to cope more readily with the changes. Try to do them all at once and you will probably give up.

Each habit will, by itself, help you to lose weight. As you build more habits in, each habit builds on the last and you will see even more progress.

Some habits will be easier to adopt than others but, at the end of the day, it is worthwhile to adopt all of them.

Eventually, when you have adopted all the habits, you will be living at the next level – you'll be healthier and more energetic in ways that you have never been before.

Read the book slowly, I have written out an action plan for each habit to make it easy for you.

No more excuses – let's dive right in!

Morning Habit #1

The MOST Common Habit of Healthy People

The most common habit of healthy people is that they wake up early every morning. Your body will thank you for it – our bodies were designed to sleep when it is nighttime and to be awake during the day when the sun is up. Getting up earlier, around the time the sun rises, is more in sync with our natural circadian rhythms.

You will find that you settle into this sleep cycle a lot easier as time goes by, resulting in the right amounts of rest each night.

The Leptin and Ghrelin Issue

Remember the last time you got to bed too late and woke up feeling less than refreshed.

Perhaps it was last night? How hungry did you feel? How easy was it to make healthy eating choices or did you just want to eat everything in sight?

Better sleep leaves you more able to deal with the stresses of the day. By not getting enough sleep, you are putting stress on your body and more cortisol is produced.

More cortisol means two of the hormones that help regulate appetite – Leptin and Ghrelin – begin to function ineffectively.

Not only are you more vulnerable to poor eating choices because you are tired, but your brain is not getting the right hunger messages from the hormones that it should.

Your brain is demanding energy and wants high calorie foods to satisfy it. Ghrelin is suppressed so the brain is not sent the message that you have eaten enough.

When you get enough sleep, your brain does not have this need for instant energy since your cortisol levels are a lot more stable. You will therefore find it a lot easier to follow a healthier eating plan and make good choices.

Even your metabolic rate benefits – those who get enough sleep have a much stronger metabolism.

According to [this article](#) in Women's Health magazine, studies have proven conclusively that being exposed to morning light by waking up earlier is linked to a decreased chance of being overweight.

Try it yourself – go to bed tonight with your curtains open and let the sun wake you in the morning.

I'm a Night Owl

This may seem a little tough at first, especially for the night owls, but it won't take long before you get used to it.

It was even hard for me at first! But what you do need to realize is that you are doing this so that you can live life to the fullest.

I figured that it came down to a simple choice – either I was happy being overweight and could carry on hitting the snooze button or I was willing to feel miserable for a few days so that I could feel great for the rest of my life.

Basically, you need to figure out whether or not the payoff for staying up late and waking up late is really worth not giving this its best chance.

ACTION PLAN

1. This is best started immediately. If you have a big day coming up or are worried about being tired, schedule it to start over a weekend instead.

2. Decide on what time is early in your part of the world and count back 8 hours from there. This is your new target bedtime.

3. About an hour before bedtime, you want to switch off your laptop, TV and cell phone. If possible, dim the lights in the house. (If you don't have a dimmer, wear a pair of sunglasses – yes, seriously!) Artificial light is very stimulating to the brain and interferes with your body's production of melatonin – the hormone that makes you sleepy.

4. Do something relaxing leading up to bedtime like reading a book – just not a best seller.

5. Go to bed when you are feeling sleepy – if you do not fall asleep within about 15 minutes either get up and start

reading again (don't forget the sunglasses) or, if you are able to, just relax in bed. It is important not to get caught up in how much sleep you are getting.

6. Set the alarm early and disable the snooze button.

7. When the alarm goes off, jump out of bed, open your curtains and bask in the sunlight. If possible, go outside for five minutes as well.

Discover Scientifically-Proven "Shortcuts" & "Hacks" to Lose Weight FASTER (With Very Little Effort)

For this month only, you can get Linda's best-selling & most popular book absolutely free – *Weight Loss Secrets You NEED to Know.*

Get Your FREE Copy Here:
TopFitnessAdvice.com/Bonus

Discover scientifically-proven tips to help you lose weight faster and easier than ever before. With this book, readers were able to improve their weight loss results and fitness levels. So, it's highly recommended that you get this book, especially while it's free!

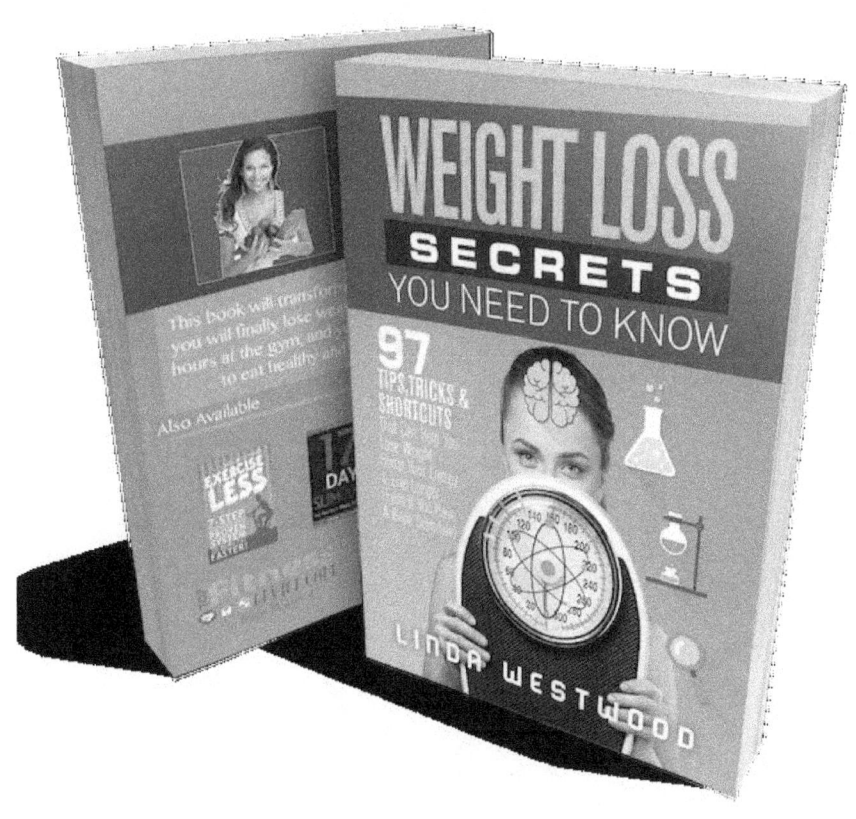

Get Your FREE Copy Here:

TopFitnessAdvice.com/Bonus

Morning Habit #2

The Morning Drink That Will Change Your Life

The next one is super easy. Drink warm lemon water first thing in the morning – use water that is tepid, not boiling, and use fresh lemons.

The Benefits

- **Smoother Digestion**

    Because of its chemical make-up, it stimulates the liver into producing bile – the acid that we need for digestion. This benefits the digestive tract even further by helping to get rid of internal toxins. Contrary to popular belief, lemon is not acidic in the digestive tract and can help treat heartburn, bloating and belching. For those with dread diseases, lemon water can help to gently get their bowel movements back on track.

- **Detoxifier/Diuretic**

    Part of the reason that it is a valuable detoxifier is that it is a diuretic – you may urinate more allowing your body to get rid of toxins faster. This also benefits your urinary tract. It doesn't stop there – it also helps to detoxify the liver.

- **Weight Loss**

    The pectin in lemons is a fiber and this is great for killing hunger pangs. Those who eat a diet that is richer in fiber, and thus richer in alkaline, actually find it easier to lose weight.

- **Boost Your Immune System**

    The high Vitamin C content makes them valuable in treating and preventing colds and flu. The high potassium content helps with the brain and nerves and also with regulating blood pressure. The Vitamin C also has anti-inflammatory effects. Overall, they are great weapons in the fight against disease.

- **Alkaline Properties**

    As mentioned before, lemon juice becomes alkaline in the blood stream. Drink it often and the blood's pH becomes less acidic. This, in turn, helps to protect you against diseases, as they require an acidic pH to thrive. If you have gout, lemon juice can help neutralize it.

- **Glowing Skin**

    Nutritional content of the juice helps to nourish the skin and also helps to fight of free radicals. It could also help fight the bacteria that cause acne. With less toxins circulating in your system, you can expect clearer skin as well. It is a well-known fact that the citrus oils in aromatherapy are stimulating. Whilst the smell of the juice in the water is not as intense, it can still give you a bit of a mood-enhancing boost.

The juice also helps to kill off the bacteria in the mouth that cause problems. That said, the acidity in the lemon can affect the tooth enamel so you should rinse out your mouth after drinking it and wait a while before brushing your teeth.

The water helps to up your hydration levels thereby increasing your energy levels. It is a great way to brush the cobwebs of sleep from your brain.

This is such an easy fix that it is amazing that it does actually work. Grow your own lemon tree if you can – that way you have fresh fruit on demand all the time.

ACTION PLAN

1. You will need half a fresh lemon a day, so unless you have a lemon tree in your garden, get a few. (No more than 4 – they are better fresh).

2. As soon as you have said hello to the sun, pour yourself a glass of tepid water – not too hot or too cold, just right!

3. Cut your lemon in half and reserve one half for tomorrow. Squeeze as much juice as you can manage from the other one.

4. Bottoms up! I find that downing it is best. I have a sweet tooth so I didn't enjoy it at first – you quickly get used to it. Now I can feel the difference if I skip my lemon water.

Morning Habit #3

Get Your Blood Flowing

Okay... now... stretch!

Do it right now – raise your hands above your head as far as you can. Feels good, doesn't it? Our bodies were born to move – it is essential for all the systems in our body.

Chances are that you don't move enough – for one, you're reading this book on improving your health and secondly, very few of us actually do.

Imagine our ancient ancestors – the stereo-typical knuckle dragging cavemen.

Do you think that he hopped out of bed, prepared his breakfast and then went off to sit at his desk? Back then, there were no desks, there was no "breakfast".

Your good old caveman got up and went out in search of food – he had to be a lean, mean hunting machine or find edible plants if he wanted to eat. He also had to be pretty fast not to get eaten himself. He spent most of his day up and about.

Nowadays, the closest most of us get to hunting is for bargains at the mall and looking for the parking spot closest to the entrance.

We all need to move more - so now we are going to incorporate stretching into our day – it will get your blood circulating and your lymphatic system up and ready for action. The proper functioning of the lymphatic system relies on us being active – if you are sluggish, so is your lymphatic system. This will speed up the removal of toxins from your body and this will help you to feel better.

Better circulation and toxin drainage will leave you looking younger and will help to prevent the formation of cellulite. The appearance of any cellulite that is there already will also improve.

It will help you to relax. Stretching your muscles is a great way to release built-up tension and to create a longer, smoother muscle shape. Your skin will start to glow and you will start to look more toned. Stretching will not build new muscle tissue but it will help tone the current muscle tissue that you have.

Do this experiment quickly – measure your tummy at its widest point. Now suck it in as far as you can and measure again. From my widest point, I could "magically" lose around 7cm around my tummy, just by sucking it in.

In effect, all I was really doing was tensing the surrounding muscles. It just goes to show how important it is to keep your muscles toned. And my tummy isn't the only flabby region on my body.

It also aids in maintaining flexibility and movement in later life. The more supple your joints and the more efficient your lymphatic system is, the higher your chances of beating diseases like rheumatism and arthritis.

If you are planning to do a workout, your body is primed. If not your whole body benefits anyway. It's win-win.

ACTION PLAN

1. Start with preparation now. Look around online for some basic stretching exercises. The Sun Salutation, used in Yoga, is a pretty good one and stretches the entire body. You should aim to stretch for at least 5 minutes.

2. All you really need is yourself and space to stretch. If you need to make space, do this tonight and then you are all ready.

3. After drinking your lemon juice, start stretching.

4. Stretching is easy, you can even do it in your PJ's – in fact the looser the clothing the better it is.

5. Do concentrate on getting the form right – take time to get into the right position. Hurrying or getting the pose wrong can do more harm than good.

6. Do try to stretch as much as you can manage but not to the point of pain. If this is painful, something is wrong.

I hope that you are enjoying this book so far, and if you could spare 30 seconds, I would greatly appreciate you leaving a review on Amazon.com.

Morning Habit #4

Start Moving ASAP

You knew this one was coming – why did you think I started with waking up earlier in the morning?

Now we are going to add a cardio workout.

Why Exercise Now?

Cardio on an empty stomach is good for you and really kicks your body into a fat-burning mode.

Studies have shown that people who exercise in the morning are more likely to stay with the exercise program and lose more weight than those that wait until later in the day.

It makes sense - the later you leave it in the day, the more chance there is that something will come up and you'll cancel.

People also have a tendency to think that one mistake makes the whole day or even week a write-off and so may delay restarting exercise and may cheat on their diets.

Get exercise done before you've had your breakfast and coffee (you may not even need the coffee anymore!).

Exercise boosts your levels of energy and gets your blood pumping – it's better than coffee and healthier too.

If You Haven't Exercised in A While

You don't have to run a marathon – if you haven't exercised for a while, walk around the garden or block a couple of times. Increase the amount of exercise you do until you are doing at least 15-30 minutes of cardio in the morning.

All cardio really means is to get your heart rate up. You want to exercise hard enough that you are breathing heavily but not so hard that you cannot also carry a conversation. You don't need any special equipment – walking at a brisk pace is cardio.

If you really don't feel like doing any cardio, just force yourself to do two minutes. If you really don't want to carry on after that, you can stop but you will usually find that starting is all the energy you need to get over that initial lag.

You'll be amazed at how fast your body starts to get used to this new regimen – remember, your body wants to move, it wants what it was designed to do.

Also, believe it or not, as your body gets used to the exercise, you'll be able to go on for longer. Your body will start to reward you with endorphins.

The mind is very powerful.

Did you know that a runner who is running 1km will start to tire as they near that mark? That same runner, at the same fitness level, if they set out to do a 10km run, will not even notice the 1km mark.

I'm not saying that you can go out and run a marathon. What I am saying is that you have more capability when it comes to exercise than you may realize.

Do take some time to find something that you enjoy doing. I remember once doing a "beginner" aerobics class – I hated it. Halfway through I was convinced I would die. I actually faked an injury to get out of it. Walking, however, was something that I could manage and that I enjoyed.

Why Cardio Will Save Your Life

It is a great outlet for stress relief – remember our caveman friend from before? When he was stressed, it meant that he had to either run away or fight his way out of it. His body physically prepared him for this by upping the amount of cortisol and adrenalin in the blood. He actually needed to respond to survive.

Nowadays, the body's response is the same but we react very differently. We seldom face the life-threatening situations that the stress reaction was designed for. The cortisol just hangs around in our blood and disrupts the rest of our hormones.

Repeated stress leads to even more disruption and the big downside of cortisol is that is causes the body to pack on visceral fat – the fat that sticks around our internal organs and causes that characteristic apple shape – the fat that is most dangerous to our health and most difficult to shift.

High levels of abdominal fat have been linked to Insulin Resistance, Type II Diabetes and Cardiovascular Disease. This cannot be stressed highly enough – that spare tire around your middle is killing you.

All it takes to keep your body happy is 30 minutes of cardio a day (you can take Sundays off, if you really want to). You don't even have to do it all at once – break it up into 10-minute chunks if that makes it easier.

Are you seriously going to sit there and tell me you can't spare 10 minutes here or there to save your life?

Is Cardio Enough?

Cardio, on its own, can only go so far. You are going to need to incorporate some strength training as well. Remember how I said that stretching didn't build muscle, it only toned them? Strength training is necessary to increase your muscle mass.

Hulk Smash!

A lot of ladies get worried when they hear the "M" word – they think by building muscle they are going to turn into a huge, muscly monster. There is nothing to worry about – building that kind of muscle takes a lot more work, heavy weights and a very specialized diet, plus hormones that women don't naturally have.

Women are also not built the same way as men, so bulking up is not as easy for us. You want to keep the weights low and the reps high and you will quickly trim some of that flab.

Women also lose muscle mass as they age. As a result, you are bound to start gaining about 2.5kg per year from the age of 35 onwards, even if nothing else changes, simply because your muscle mass will decrease.

Weight bearing exercise is essential to stave off this loss and the consequent "middle age spread", and also to help prevent osteoporosis.

Men and Women Now

Muscle burns more calories at rest than fat does. Muscle works harder – fat is lazy.

Which would you rather have in your corner? Two to three good sessions of strength training is really all you need.

Do take some time to learn how to properly work the different muscle groups – as with stretching, if you get it wrong, you won't like the results.

There are many tutorials on the web, books and exercise DVDs that can help you with this. You do not have to buy expensive specialized equipment. A simple set of dumbbells will be sufficient.

You should also allow your body some rest time between workouts so that it can repair the tissue. Essentially you are tearing the muscle tissue with the workout – when the body builds it back, it builds it back stronger.

If you want to do some strength training every day, you can – just don't work the same muscle groups two days in a row.

ACTION PLAN

1. If you are currently very unfit or on medication, have a chat with your doctor first about suitable exercises for you.

2. Do some research about cardio exercises and strength training and find something that you find appealing. There are tons of exercise DVDs that you can use in the comfort and privacy of your own home.

3. After stretching, change into your workout clothes if necessary, and get going.

4. Get started and commit to exercising every day – even just for 10 minutes. Slow and steady wins the race.

Morning Habit #5

The BIGGEST Mistake Most People Make in The Morning

Most people skip breakfast. This is the worst health and dieting mistake that you could possibly make.

EAT BREAKFAST!

Your body needs the nourishment after the workout or it can't get to repairing itself. You have to eat breakfast in order to help boost your metabolism for the rest of the day.

Think about it – if you ate dinner at 7pm and eat nothing again until 12:00 pm you are going 17 hours without food – in most parts of the world going without food for that long is considered starving.

Worse still, your body will feel that it is starving and you will actually eat more than you should at lunch and dinner.

According to <u>a study conducted by the IFT</u>, those that skip breakfast are more likely to weigh more than those that do not and are more likely to have other bad eating habits as well.

It was found that those who skipped breakfast were more likely to choose calorie-rich food and sugary sodas as opposed to healthier options such as fruit and vegetables.

It's What You Eat That Counts

You don't have to eat a huge plate of food either – just make sure that you eat the right foods. Get creative – you want healthy food, not boring food.

What about an olive omelet or smoked salmon on rye bread? Why not have some veggies with your meal?

Protein Please

You need to have at least one serving of high-quality protein with every meal – breakfast included. Protein will help you feel fuller for longer and is essential for muscle repair and energy production.

Choose whatever protein you like – yoghurt is a good choice, tastes good and is filling. A small tub of yoghurt is quite a good idea. The only caveat is that you need to get the natural, unsweetened type. It can be full fat but must not have any sugar in it. You can pulse up some frozen berries or chop in some fruit to make it taste better if you like.

If you want some bacon, go for it – just remember that a serving of bacon is two slices, no more than that – even if it is back bacon. Consider grilling your bacon in the oven, it is a lot easier and healthier that way.

In fact, here's another time saving breakfast tip. Take a muffin pan and spray with nonstick spray. Break an egg into one of the compartments. Repeat in another compartment if you want two eggs. Season this with cayenne pepper and a little salt. Place your two rashers side by side over another compartment and bake in at 180 degrees Celsius for about 15-20 minutes. Stick it in before you have your lemon water and it will be ready to eat when you are finished exercising.

You could also opt for some cheese on your toast if you want – again, don't go overboard – get out your potato peel and peel off some cheese as though you were peeling potatoes – thin slices. You can have up to nine thin slices of a regular sized block of cheese.

I'm Going to Egg You On

Eggs are a great source of protein and easy to prepare – what I normally do is to boil four or five at a time. I have one or two at breakfast, depending on how hungry I am. It's easy, it's ready when I need it and there are no excuses for not eating breakfast.

The old "eggs causing cholesterol" myth has now finally been debunked. Eat the egg, eat the yolk – it is nature's super food.

You Need Some Carbs as Well

Low carb diets are popular but even the proponent's stress low-carb, not no-carb.

Add in one serving of complex carbohydrates – this helps your body recover after your workout and ensures that you have an even spike of energy to last you through to lunch.

Oatmeal is a good option. No sugar! You can add in some raisins or fruit or mix it with your yoghurt to make it taste better.

Whole-wheat toast is another. You want carbs that will provide steady energy so check for carbs that fall on the low side of the GI scale.

A Serving of Fat Please

Fat is good again! Do stick to natural, unprocessed fats though. Yes, you can have some real butter on your toast or in your oatmeal.

Otherwise why not have a bit of avocado? Half an avocado is one serving size and it makes a killer spread for toast.

Olives and avocados are a super healthy form of fat – monounsaturated.

Studies have shown that one serving of monounsaturated fat with each meal helps you to lose belly fat and improves your cardiovascular health.

I always have one form of monounsaturated fat with my breakfast. Servings are easy to remember - about 12 nuts or half an avocado or 10 olives.

Smoothies

If you really can't handle a solid breakfast, a smoothie is a good substitute. I enjoy them because you can sneak all sorts of healthy things in there and not taste them. This is one of my favorite recipes.

Ingredients

- 1 cup almond milk
- 1 banana or apple
- 1 cup frozen berries
- 175ml tub of plain yoghurt
- 1 carrot
- 1 tablespoon turmeric
- 1 teaspoon cinnamon
- 1 half teaspoon cayenne pepper
- 1 tablespoon pumpkin seeds

Method

1. I just whizz it all up and enjoy it. It makes quite a bit so I put some in a thermos for a mid-morning snack. The turmeric has a nice smooth flavor and you barely taste the cayenne pepper. This gives me energy all day.

Spice it Up

With the smoothie recipe, you may have been a little thrown with the mention of turmeric. This is actually a wonderful spice that is very popular in India. It is great at treating inflammation and the active ingredient, curcumin, has been found to be as effective an analgesic as aspirin.

It is a traditional Indian remedy for treating acid indigestion and heartburn. About a tablespoon daily is enough. Take my advice though and don't take it on an empty stomach. Mix it into your smoothie, cook with it or mix it into a half a glass of milk.

Plain oatmeal can take a bit of getting used to – boost the flavor by adding some cinnamon.

Cinnamon has been shown to be an effective stabilizer of blood sugar and a valuable ally in the fight against insulin resistance and Type II Diabetes. It is this effect that makes it such a valuable weight loss tool. It has been proven to be as effective in some cases as prescribed diabetes medication. Adding a teaspoon of cinnamon a day is all that is needed to see benefits.

Cayenne Pepper has been proven to stimulate the metabolism, help clear away plaque in the arteries and to help reduce levels of LDL cholesterol (the one you don't want). By stimulating your metabolism, it helps you to lose more weight.

In fact, all members of the chili family will help to rev up metabolism and speed up weight loss.

Ginger is known to soothe an upset stomach but can also be instrumental when it comes to weight loss – it boosts your metabolism and can work to suppress your appetite as well.

Cardamom is not really a spice that one sees used much outside of curries but this is a pity as it is believed that it can boost the burning of fat within your body.

One of My Easy Breakfasts

I really don't enjoy cooking so I will often soak my oatmeal overnight in water – that way it is ready to eat in the morning. I sprinkle some cinnamon over the top of it and mix in some natural yogurt. I finish it off with a chopped apple or banana and some flaked almonds.

ACTION PLAN

1. Plan ahead – read up some more about low-GI foods and research some breakfast ideas that appeal to you.

2. Do any prep work that you can the night before – I will get together all the ingredients that I need for the smoothie and measure them out ready for the next morning. NO excuses. Make it as easy as possible to make your breakfast.

3. After your workout finish preparing your breakfast.

4. Sit down and enjoy.

5. Take some time to eat – try not to eat on the run unless you have to.

Morning Habit #6

Stack Your Breakfast With THIS

Pile on the protein at breakfast.

Do you want to lose weight? Do you want maximum energy? Do you want enhanced mental function all day? If the answer to any of these questions is yes, you need to eat a big portion of protein for breakfast. More protein with fewer carbs or no carbs at all is what you should be aiming for, especially if you are trying to build muscle.

In a study published in 2011 in the medical journal, Obesity, it was found that those who ate a high protein breakfast felt satiated for much longer during the day, had far fewer cravings and less instances of late-night snacking. They lost more weight than the control group as well and reported feeling sharper and more alert.

The Very Best Protein Bet

I have already extolled the wonders of having eggs with breakfast but this does bear repeating. Eggs are the most nutrient dense and complete foods on the planet.

Think about it for a second – that egg is designed to feed a chicken embryo and help it grow big and strong.

All that goodness is contained in the yolk – if you are throwing out the yolk you are missing out on:

- Iron
- Calcium
- Phosphorus
- Thiamin
- Zinc
- Folate
- Vitamin B6
- Vitamin B12
- Vitamin A
- Vitamin D
- Vitamin E
- Omega 3 Fatty Acids
- Essential Amino Acids

Eggs are high in the good kind of cholesterol, but that is NOT a bad thing – our body produces its own cholesterol anyway, so by eating it we actually short-circuit the production of the bad cholesterol.

In controlled studies to measure the impact of eggs on weight loss, participants were instructed to eat up to three eggs a day.

At the end of the study it was found that those who ate the eggs lost more weight, had lower inflammation levels and also reduced levels of cholesterol.

Scientists did have a cautionary note though – there are some indications that diabetics and those that have a family history of hypercholesterolemia should eat no more than an egg a day at most. More research is needed but if either of these conditions apply to you, it is better to err on the side of caution.

Alternatives to Eggs

Not everyone wants to eat eggs every day so here are some other alternatives:

- **Meat is back! Meat is good! Yes, even red meat!**

    For years we have been told that saturated fats are bad for us. New scientific evidence actually points to the exact opposite – they are good for us. It is the hydrogenated or trans-fats that are the problem.

    So every time you have a barbeque put on an extra chop or steak and have it with your breakfast the next day. You'll find that you have stable energy throughout the day and will all be able to concentrate better. You also won't fixate on food as much either.

- **Nuts and Seeds**

    All you need is 75g of nuts a day to see the benefits. Eat them over and above your normal protein intake and you'll get a healthy boost. They are calorie dense but it should be remembered that they contain loads of nutrients and monounsaturated fats. Nuts will also help you feel full, give you an energy boost and keep your blood levels more stable.

- **Lentils, Chickpeas and Quinoa**

These are all high protein foods that are great if you are a vegetarian or want something different.

ACTION PLAN

1. Think about how you can incorporate more protein in your breakfast starting tomorrow. Protein is very filling so you should consider cutting down the carb content.

2. Make it easy for yourself – boil a few eggs to keep for tomorrow and the next day – hardboiled eggs will store well in the fridge for a couple of days.

3. Reconsider dinner portions as well – cook extra meat so that you have some for breakfast.

4. In the morning, after you have exercised, eat breakfast as usual but with the added protein.

Once again, thank you for reading this book, and I hope you're getting a lot of valuable information. I would greatly appreciate it if you could take 30 seconds to leave me a review for this book on Amazon.com.

Morning Habit #7

A Morning Fat Burning Boost

Drink a cup of green tea in the morning. Green tea is the best health drink that there is. It is high in anti-oxidants and other nutrients and will help to, amongst other things, increase the amount of fat lost, reduce your risk of developing cancer and increase the level at which your brain functions as well.

There are a host of benefits – we do nowhere near fully understand everything that green tea can do. But here I will list the benefits that have been scientifically proven:

Health Improving Compounds Abound in Green Tea

A lot of the bioactive compounds survive the process from tea leave to teacup. The most important of these are the antioxidants. Antioxidants help to prevent free radicals forming. Fewer free radicals mean less damage to your system. You will not appear to age as fast and will be less likely to pick up diseases.

Cancer is still one of the biggest killers of our age. It has now been established that damage caused by oxidation is a big contributor when it comes to the growth of cancerous cells. Oxidation is caused by free radicals and these can be neutralized by antioxidants. For maximum protection, skip the milk – milk lowers the number of antioxidants present.

Adult onset diabetes has now been rated a global epidemic and affects hundreds of millions of people. The disease is characterized by high levels of blood sugar and the inability of the body to cope because insulin effectiveness is reduced.

Green tea has been shown to help improve the body's sensitivity to insulin and to lower the levels of sugar in the blood. A study in Japan found that you could decrease you chances of developing Adult Onset Diabetes by as much as 42%. Studies show that green tea can improve insulin sensitivity and reduce blood sugar

Cardiovascular diseases are the biggest mass murderers the world has seen. Green tea reduces your risk of being a victim by improving your statistics where it matters – your LDL cholesterol, overall cholesterol and triglyceride levels. Because of the antioxidant abilities of green tea, LDL cholesterol is less likely to become oxidized. This is a big one when it comes to cardiovascular disease. Drinking green tea regularly, without milk, reduces your chances of cardiovascular disease by as much as 31%.

Catechins have anti-bacterial and anti-viral actions as well. This is good news for your teeth – the tea can decrease the growth rate of the plaque-forming bacteria in the mouth. It also helps fight bad breath.

Your Brain on Green Tea

There is caffeine in green tea so it will make you more alert – the amount is not quite as high as that found in coffee so you won't get the jitters either. Caffeine actually makes you more alert by blocking Adenosine – a neurotransmitter with that has an inhibitory effect. Because it blocks Adenosine, more neurons in the brain fire and there are higher concentrations of neurotransmitters like Norepinephrine and Dopamine.

Caffeine will improve your mood, make you more alert, increase your response times and boost your memory. Green tea has something the coffee doesn't though – L-Theanine, the amino acid that is able to make its way across the barrier between blood and brain.

This amino acid causes an increase in the activity of GABA – the neurotransmitter that helps with calming us. Alpha waves in the brain increase in number and you become calmer but more focused at the same time.

Studies have been conducted on the effect of caffeine together with L-Theanine and it has been found that each works together to increase the beneficial effects of the other. You will have the energy to do what you need to do and also feel better overall – with no jittery crashes when the caffeine wears off. Sticking to your diet plan is easier to do the increased levels of dopamine in the brain.

The long-term benefits of drinking green tea are also pretty impressive. Parkinson's and Alzheimer's are two of the most common dementia-related diseases today. Promising studies indicate that it is the compound called catechins in the tea that could help to protect the neuron action in the brain, thereby reducing the chances of developing these diseases.

Lose Weight

Take any of those "miracle" weight loss pills off the shelf and check the ingredients. I'm willing to bet that at least 80% contain green tea. That is because, controlled trials have proven that the tea does rev up your body's ability to burn fat and also increases your metabolism. You may burn as much as 4% more energy and experience as much as 17% more when it comes to the oxidation of fat.

The caffeine boosts your performance physically because of the way that it moves fatty acids out of the fat cells and thus makes it possible for them to be used by the body as fuel.

Separate reviews have concluded that caffeine, on average, will improve performance physically by as much as 12%.

Given the metabolic boost green tea gives, its sensible to assume that it will help with weight loss. Studies have proven that this conclusion is correct. You lose body fat, particularly stubborn belly fat.

ACTION PLAN

1. Go to the store and get some green tea.

2. The choice between tea bags and tea leaves is a personal one and the studies haven't indicated that there is any difference in results. Personally, I prefer tea bags – they're less messy.

3. Either way, make it as you would normal tea. Allow it to brew for at least 5 minutes for the full effect.

4. Add a little honey if you want for flavor. Personally though, I think it tastes fine as is.

5. Sip slowly.

6. The used teabags are great for the compost heap so dispose of them by tossing them in there.

Morning Habit #8

The Crucial Habit to Weight Loss Success

Weigh yourself in the morning!

There is a lot of information out there on the Internet and in the media about how you should only weigh yourself once a week so that you aren't as obsessed with your weight.

Like you forget about it all week until you weigh in...

I tried weighing myself once a week. It didn't work. The first week was fine. I weighed myself on Sunday morning, wrote the weight down and then went around stealing furtive glances at my scale from time to time.

The second week went pretty badly. To be honest, I only remembered to weight myself again on Wednesday. I let it go on for a few more weeks and then went back to daily weigh-ins.

It is easier to remember to weigh yourself daily - you get into the habit of weighing yourself.

The key is to weigh yourself at the same time EVERY MORNING – that is the only true way to keep track of how you are progressing. I find it's easiest to weight myself as soon as I get out of bed.

That way, you have no excuses about having eaten something "heavy" or having had too many cups of tea. Your weight will fluctuate throughout the day and may even fluctuate from day to day.

If you want an accurate of your progress, you must weigh yourself at the same time every day, when your body is in a similar state to what it was before.

The other reason why weighing yourself daily is important is that it is quite motivating. Whilst we know intellectually that the movement on the scale is not necessarily indicative of weight loss, you do start to see patterns after tracking for at least a week.

You'll know straight away if something has gone seriously wrong with the plan, instead of only finding out three or four days later and doing even more damage.

You'll be more inclined to "behave" if you've weighed yourself in the morning. Either the results will be motivating because you pick up losses straight away or you get scared straight because you've been bad.

It's a win-win.

ACTION PLAN

1. An electronic scale is more accurate and weighs parts of kilograms as well. If you do not have one, try and get one.

2. Start showing your scale some love. Dust it off and put is somewhere that you'll notice it first thing in the morning.

3. Do make sure that the scale is on a level surface.

4. Don't put it where you can stub your toe or injure yourself – scales can be hard on toes.

5. Download a fitness app that allows you to track your weight. I personally like "Calorie Counter" by FatSecret. It is free and easy to use and it never forgets - I have stats going back two years on there. There is a whole lot more it can do but I usually use it for weigh-ins. You can choose to use it on your phone, tablet or PC. It syncs between devices as well.

6. Alternatively, go old-school and buy a notepad to record the results.

7. It is important to write them down immediately or you will forget. It's not so hard to remember that you weigh 85kg, for example. But is it 85.6kg or 85.8?

8. Yes, the differences matter!

Enjoying this book?

Check out my other best sellers!

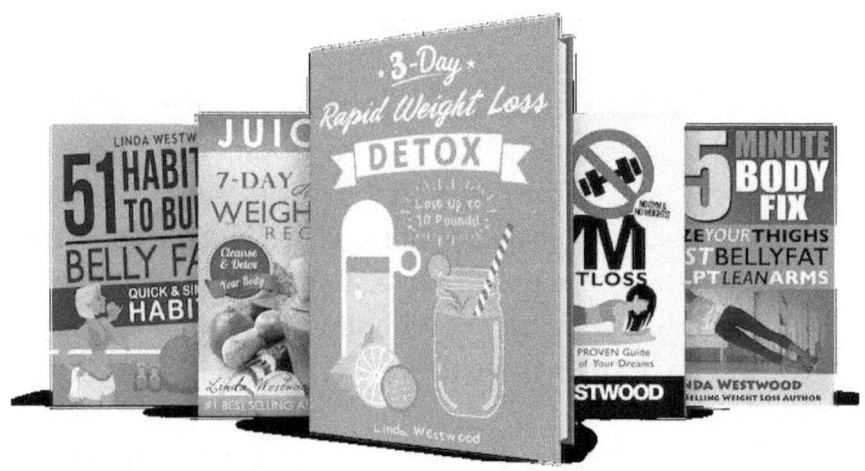

Get your next book on sale here:

TopFitnessAdvice.com/go/books

Morning Habit #9

The ONLY Pill That You Should Take

Take a daily multivitamin every morning with breakfast. You do not need to take so many supplements that you rattle, but you do need a multivitamin. Our diets simply no longer provide enough nutrients to keep us optimally healthy. Taking a multivitamin every morning at the same time is a great way to make a habit of it and a great way to keep the nutrient levels in your body constant. This is great news if you are trying to lose weight…

Nutrient deficiencies lead to cravings for foods that the body believes will best fit its needs. The body is not all that clever at judging what is good for it – if it wants energy, it will not choose a nice juicy apple but will rather go for the instant rush of sugary foods.

The body can be quite a bully when it wants to be – it is going to be hard to withstand the cravings. It is harder when your body is screaming for nutrients. It is virtually impossible if you are stressed out.

Contrary to popular belief, taking a multi-vitamin is not going to increase your appetite. Studies have actually shown that those taking a multivitamin reported feeling fuller than those taking the placebo.

Scientists believe that even slight nutrient deficiencies, whilst not escalating into full-blown cravings, may cause us to eat more. Then, of course, there are natural minerals that are very hard for us to get but that are very beneficial when it comes to weight loss.

Chromium is one such mineral - Chromium Piconlinate to be precise. Supplementation with this mineral has been found to be as effective as controlling blood sugar in people with insulin resistance as conventional drugs.

If you are on diabetes meds, talk to your doctor before starting ANY supplementation. You MUST also monitor your blood sugar daily to see if there is an improvement. Do NOT go off your meds without talking to your doctor first!

Aside from the weight loss benefits associated with taking supplements, there are proven health benefits as well.

Modern living takes a lot out of us and supplementation will help your body to cope with the stress and function at optimal levels again.

The B vitamins, for example, help you to deal with excessive stress. Vitamin C is important for your immune system. Vitamin D, something that most of us are lacking in, is vital for fighting inflammation and oxidative stress. The list goes on and on...

The key, though, is to take the vitamins in the right quantities and proportions. Mega-dosing is, at best, an expensive and useless exercise and, at worst, dangerous.

When you take mega-doses of the water-soluble vitamins, the body takes what it needs at the time and flushes the rest out of your system. When you take mega-doses of fat-soluble vitamins, the excess is stored in the fat tissues and toxicity can develop - yet another thing to thank your fat for!

Take your supplements in the morning - that is when your body needs them most. It also helps the body to make optimal use of the supplements.

It is important to concentrate on quality. Cheaper brands have binding agents and fillers that may not be so good for you.

ACTION PLAN

1. Do some research and find a good supplement available in your area. Ask your doctor or pharmacist for advice.

2. Don't be swayed by the advertising. Compare the supplements according to their nutritional content and what preservatives and binders are used.

3. Be careful about buying in bulk – make sure that you will be able to use all the vitamins before the bottle expires.

4. Store your vitamins in a dry, dark cupboard.

5. Take the required dose straight after breakfast, with some plain water.

Others who are considering purchasing this book would love to know what you think. If you could spare a few seconds, they would greatly appreciate reading an honest review from you. Simply visit the page on Amazon.com.

Morning Habit #10

Boost Your Fiber Intake

Take a fiber supplement in the morning with your breakfast. It does not matter whether or not this is in pill form or as a drink. You are probably not getting all the fiber that you need from your diet, especially not if you eat a lot of refined foods.

Fiber supplement that contain psyllium (like Metamucil and Konsyl) are safe for every day use. Fiber is essential if you want to lose weight and maintain the weight loss. If you are not getting enough fiber, you can have as much as 4-8lbs of undigested food sluggishly moving around in your intestines.

There are beneficial bacteria in the colon that help us to digest the food and get all the goodness we can from it. Without enough fiber, the "bad" bacteria soon overrun these good little soldiers.

Instead of the nutrients being taken out of the food, it literally rots in your gut. This causes gas to develop and you start bloating. Your body does not get the nutrients it needs so you are hungrier and eat more. The whole cycle starts again.

The rotting food is not only causing you troubles with your weight though – toxins released by the fermentation process are being absorbed into your blood stream and putting you at risk for serious health issues.

There are two types of fiber – soluble and insoluble. We need both. The body can digest soluble fiber and it helps to mop up the dangerous LDL cholesterol in your blood and helps to keep blood sugar levels in check.

The body does not absorb insoluble fiber but it helps keep the food moving at a steady pace through the digestive tract. It also helps you feel fuller faster.

Think about it for a second. How many oranges can you eat in one sitting – imagine that they are your favorite food – before you feel full?

Now take the fiber away – like they do when they make orange juice.

Did you know that to get one cup of pure orange juice, you need to squeeze 22 oranges? That is not cost effective for the makers of the juice though so they dilute it with denatured juice and add sugar so it tastes better.

Your cup of orange juice is about the equivalent of eating 6 oranges with almost the same amount of sugar as you will find in a glass of coke. Take the fiber out and it is easy to get your 5 – 9 portions of fruit and vegetables a day.

The problem is that without the fiber, there is nothing to slow down the body's absorption of the sugar and your sugar levels spike. Your body also doesn't register the calories because they are liquid so it won't help you feel fuller either.

The net result is that you may as well be drinking sugar – what's left of the vitamins in that juice will never outweigh the dangerous sugar rush. At the same time though, we can't always eat the way we should. A fiber supplement makes things easier all round.

ACTION PLAN

1. Go out and buy a fiber supplement.

2. It takes time to work so you don't have to worry about embarrassing accidents at work.

3. Take it as directed every morning.

4. You can even take it with your lemon water.

5. Ideally it should be taken on an empty stomach.

6. You can expect to experience some initial discomfort – gas and more regular bowel movements are common at first.

7. The discomfort usually passes in a week or two, once your body gets into a proper digestive rhythm again.

Morning Habit #11

The MOST Important Habit in This Book

PLAN YOUR DAY.

Sit down and take a couple of minutes to plan out what you will do in during the upcoming day.

The most commonly cited reason for people not to stick to their health plan is that they were caught unawares.

If you have a plan set up, you are less likely to fail.

By planning when you'll eat, what you eat, etc., you can make sure that the resources are in place when you need them.

Planning healthy meals, snacks and activities will ensure that you don't wolf down the contents of your fridge at night because you forgot to eat lunch.

Planning for what to do when trouble strikes is good insurance as well. How will you distract yourself if a craving strikes? Make a plan every morning and hold yourself accountable for it.

Commit to it for that day – taking it one step at a time is used in recovery programs because it works. Committing to one day is a whole lot easier than committing your entire life.

ACTION PLAN

1. Think about the day ahead and what you will be doing.

2. Are there going to be any potential risks to your health plan?

3. How will you deal with them if there are?

4. When are you going to have your meals and what are you going to have to eat?

5. What other actions will you take today to improve your wellness?

6. You can write the list out if you like and sign it or you can just commit to it mentally.

Morning Habit #12

Plan to Be A Binge Drinker

Fill up your water bottle for the day ahead.

Having the water ready to drink is not only a visual reminder of how much you need to drink throughout the day but it makes it a lot easier for you as well.

If the water is in front of you, you are more likely to drink it. If you have to remember to go get it, you will probably forget.

It doesn't take long to get into the habit of drinking water and it so good for you.

If you don't like the taste of plain water, add a bit of lemon juice or some mint leaves to jazz it up a little. Always add your own flavorings. Flavored bottle water can have as much sugar in it as a can of cool drink.

Why Drink Water?

Our bodies are made up of 70% water. You can go for a couple of weeks without eating but you won't last 3 days without water. Not being adequately hydrated can makes your brain send signals to your body. The problem is that we often mistake this as hunger and eat.

A lot of the time, what you think is hunger is actually a sign of dehydration.

When your body is short on water, it hangs on to what it's got. That's why you so often lose so much weight in the first week of the diet – the body is better hydrated so it let's go of the water it has been retaining.

In fact, by the time you feel thirsty you are already in the first stages of dehydration. Being properly hydrated makes all the body's systems work well together. Your body becomes more efficient at waste disposal and your skin looks younger and plumper. There is no moisturizer out there that can compete when it comes to drinking enough water.

It's also addictive – I started on one bottle a day and I'm now on 2 liters a day. I carry my water bottle wherever I go with me and I can honestly say it is my favorite drink. I will choose it instead of cool drink nine times out of ten. I love it plain and just out of the tap.

You actually become quite the connoisseur – I have my favorite brands of bottled water now.

Once you get used to being fully hydrated, you'll wonder how you ever managed before. You'll be amazed at the results you get – I haven't had a urinary tract infection in over twenty years and I credit that to drinking enough water.

ACTION PLAN

1. Get yourself a bottle to drink out of now. I prefer glass bottles – they keep the water at a more even temperature and the water seems to taste better out of glass.

2. Start with a 500ml bottle of water and work your way up from there.

3. Fill it up and take it to work with you.

4. Leave it on your desk or somewhere that you can always see it.

5. Drink a glass of water whenever you remember to.

6. If it's very hot, I often put my bottle in the freezer overnight – just don't fill it completely - the water expands when frozen. When you take it out in the morning, add some water to get it to start melting - you'll have nice cold water for most of the day.

I hope you have learned something from this book so far and would greatly appreciate it if you could leave an honest review on Amazon.com.

Morning Habit #13

Make & Carry Healthy Snacks with You

Make healthy snacks for yourself throughout the day and keep them on hand. You are bound to feel hunger pangs between meals, plan ahead and have healthy snacks ready for these times.

Healthy snacking is actually great for weight loss – it balances out your blood sugar levels and gently stokes your metabolism.

Keeping your blood sugar levels constant is going to help you stick to your healthy eating plan. It is the sugar rushes from eating the wrong foods that causes the subsequent energy crash and the need to eat more.

Healthy eating is going to help keep you off sugary foods and simple carbs. Filling up on healthy food will help you to resist the siren's call of the vending machine.

ACTION PLAN

1. Make a list of healthy snacks that you can keep with you. Nuts and seeds are great ideas. Real fruit is also quite filling. Dried fruit is technically better for you then sweets but it still has too much sugar in it.

2. Watch out for snack bars that are labeled as healthy – check the ingredients, a lot of them are laden with sugar and fats.

3. If you can discipline yourself to do so, you can have a couple of PIECES of dark chocolate – not slabs, pieces. Make sure that there is at least 80% cocoa in them.

4. Olives make a nice snack.

5. Keep an emergency stash in your drawer at work at all times.

6. Make sure that you always have at least two snack packs handy all the time.

BONUS Morning Habit #14

Carb Up in the AM!

If you're going to eat carbs, eat them in the morning. You need to stick to complex carbs that release a steady stream of energy. Anything that has a G.I. of over 50 is out.

Complex carbs have three or more sugars and have a high fiber content. Simple carbs are mainly made up of two.

Sweetness is usually a fair indication of how complex the carb is. Complex carbs often taste blander, although this is not always the case.

The best way to tell is to check your energy levels and hunger after eating the carb. If you get a sudden rush of energy, it is more likely to be a simple carb. If you feel hungry again a couple of hours afterwards, despite having eaten your fill, it is definitely a simple carb.

Examples of Good Carbs

- Whole grains
- Plain oats
- Nuts, seeds
- Brown rice
- Quinoa
- Barley
- Most vegetables

The fiber content in complex carbs is what makes them so much healthier – this slows down the rate that the sugars in the carbs are absorbed into the blood stream.

They will also help you to feel full longer and they are heart healthy. If you are battling to manage on breakfast until lunch, add some complex carbs.

It is not a good idea to eat them later in the day – your body needs time to process them.

ACTION PLAN

1. What simple carbs are you eating now? Check everything that you currently eat for breakfast and see what the G.I. rating for each food is.

2. Choose from the list of healthy carbs. They should not compose more than a quarter of your daily diet.

3. Evaluate how you feel after eating them – did they give a rush of energy. Are you reaching for more a couple of hours later? If so, they are probably simple carbs.

4. Slowly try to cut carbs out of the diet. Do eat vegetables but start to cut back on grains. Current thinking is that our digestive tract cannot digest grains properly because they are a relatively new addition to our diets.

BONUS Morning Habit #15

The Only OTHER Pill That You Should Take

Take a fish oil supplement every morning with your breakfast. The alternative to supplementation is to have two servings of oily fish a week. Most of us don't get that - hence the supplement.

It has to be cod liver or fish oil because that is already in a form that the body can use. Omega-3s from plant sources are in a form that the body has to convert before it can use. The body is not very efficient when it comes to this process.

Omega-3 is what you want. Do not get pulled into the marketing hype for the other omegas. We need more Omega-3s than we do Omega-6s and you are probably getting plenty of the latter from your diet.

If your body does not get the right type of fat from its diet, it will hold on to any fat it can get. Your body can literally be morbidly obese and not have enough essential fats at the same time.

Essential fatty acids will help shift that stubborn belly fat. You will not see too much of a shift on the scale but you will find that you lose centimeters.

They help to convert bad LDL cholesterol into the healthier HDL type. They are essential to the health of your skin and the mucosal membranes in the body. Taking it at the same time every day helps to keep the levels constant – your body can use is as necessary.

Watch out for bulk offers – these oils can go rancid.

ACTION PLAN

1. Choose a good quality supplement.

2. You may have to do some experimenting with different supplement ranges. I always thought that the Omega-3 thing was a bit of a waste of time. I bought the brand that I am currently taking because it was on special. After about a month on it, I could honestly say that I felt that it was making a difference.

3. It is best to take these with meals to stop the flavor from repeating throughout the morning.

4. If you do not like fish, you are not initially going to like the fact that the flavor does repeat on you. But that will go away in time.

Don't forget to share your thoughts on this book by leaving a review on Amazon.com. It takes just a few seconds.

BONUS Morning Habit #16

Rebound to A Healthy Life

Rebound every morning for 5 minutes after waking up.

Rebounding is fun and very good for you.

Benefits

- Get the blood pumping and make you feel energized.

- Help with the circulation and drainage of lymph and toxins.

- It is good cardio exercise and is a lot easier on your body than pounding a pavement when it comes to impact stress.

- It helps to improve stamina and endurance.

- It revs up the metabolism.

- Did I mention that it's fun?

- It counts as exercise, seriously.

- You get more bang for your buck – because you are basically defying gravity, you get a more intense workout than you would from running. Five minutes on the trampoline is equivalent to about double the same time running hard.

- It's relatively quiet and doesn't take up too much space.

- The trampoline itself doesn't cost a lot – meaning no more wasted money on a gym subscription you don't use.

- You can do more than just bounce around – you can run in place, skip, jump – get creative, it will never get boring.

- There are even workout DVDs that you can get to go with it.

ACTION PLAN

1. Get yourself a mini-trampoline.

2. Place it where you'll see it first thing in the morning – maybe next to the scale.

3. Climb off your scale and onto your rebounder – before you have your lemon water or anything else.

4. Five minutes is harder than it sounds. Keep at it.

Discover Scientifically-Proven "Shortcuts" & "Hacks" to Lose Weight FASTER (With Very Little Effort)

For this month only, you can get Linda's best-selling & most popular book absolutely free – *Weight Loss Secrets You NEED to Know.*

Get Your FREE Copy Here:
TopFitnessAdvice.com/Bonus

Discover scientifically-proven tips to help you lose weight faster and easier than ever before. With this book, readers were able to improve their weight loss results and fitness levels. So, it's highly recommended that you get this book, especially while it's free!

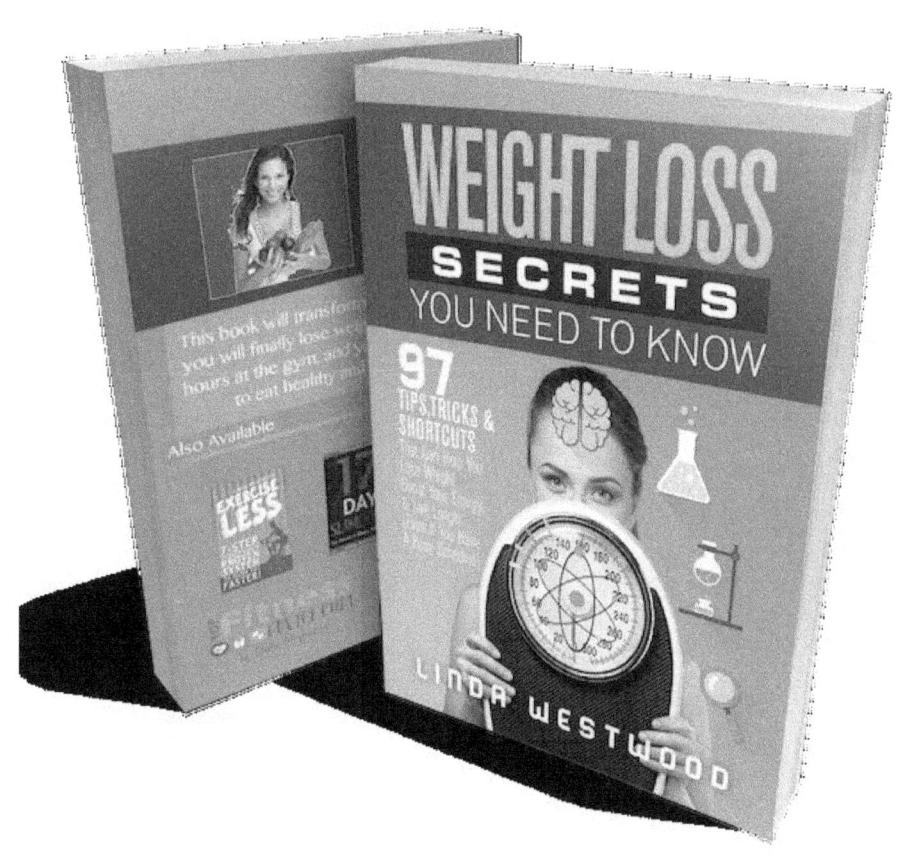

Get Your FREE Copy Here:

TopFitnessAdvice.com/Bonus

Conclusion

I can't believe that we have finally come to the end of the book. By now, you will have incorporated all of the habits and will definitely have started seeing some improvements.

Some habits would have been easier to adopt than others – do you see now what it was important not to do everything at once?

You have to admit that, on the whole, you haven't really had to do that much differently though. These were small changes to make with some really big payoffs.

I have always felt that starting your morning off in the right way sets you up for the whole day. I am sure that the healthy morning habits are now seeping through into the other parts of your life as well.

By now, most of these habits will pretty much be second nature to you.

If you want to see more progress, start adopting some of the morning principles to the rest of your day as well – eat a similarly balanced lunch and supper – protein at every meal is essential to keeping up your energy levels and weight loss.

Do increase your intake of green tea throughout the day – three to four cups is ideal.

Also, as this plan shows, you don't need to be afraid to mix things up a bit – change is good. By now you will have learned better how to listen to your body and its needs. The body can act like a naughty little kid at times but, with the right discipline, you can get it firing on all cylinders again.

You'll start to crave the healthier foods –I couldn't believe it myself when I one day started craving carrots!

Eventually, your body will start wanting you want – a healthier lifestyle. This desire was actually in the back of your mind along but your body was just being too lazy to admit it!

Do keep up to date with the latest actual scientific research and make decisions based on sound advice rather than a great marketing campaign. Thirty years ago, egg yolks were bad and margarine was good for you. Thanks to intensive marketing campaigns, there are still a lot of people who believe these myths. Always read the ingredients list before putting it in your trolley.

Now that you have overcome the hardest bit, I wish you good health and good luck!

Final Words

I would like to thank you for purchasing my book and I hope I have been able to help you and educate you on something new.

If you have enjoyed this book and would like to share your positive thoughts, could you please take 30 seconds of your time to go back and give me a review on my Amazon book page.

I greatly appreciate seeing these reviews because it helps me share my hard work.

You can leave me a review on Amazon.com.

Again, thank you and I wish you all the best!

Enjoying this book?

Check out my other best sellers!

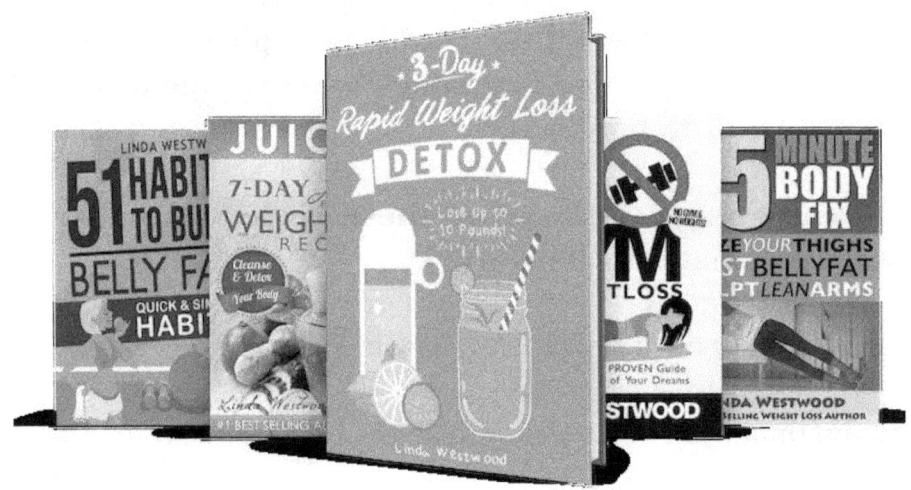

Get your next book on sale here:

TopFitnessAdvice.com/go/books

www.ingramcontent.com/pod-product-compliance
Lightning Source LLC
Chambersburg PA
CBHW031202020426
42333CB00013B/774